DR. OLIVIA H. WELLS

GOLO DIET COOKBOOK

Delicious and Nutrient- Rich Recipes for Successful Weight Loss on the GOLO Diet

Copyright © 2023 by DR. OLIVIA H. WELLS

All rights reserved. No part of this publication may be reproduced, stored or transmitted in any form or by any means, electronic, mechanical, photocopying, recording, scanning, or otherwise without written permission from the publisher. It is illegal to copy this book, post it to a website, or distribute it by any other means without permission.

First edition

This book was professionally typeset on Reedsy.
Find out more at reedsy.com

Contents

INTRODUCTION	v
BOOK DESCRIPTION	viii
INTRODUCTION TO THE GOLO DIET	1
Understanding the GOLO Diet: A Science-based Approach to Weight Loss	1
Benefits of the GOLO Diet for Long-term Health and Well-being	4
GETTING STARTED WITH THE GOLO DIET	7
Essential Principles and Guidelines for Success	7
GOLO Diet Phases: Transitioning and Maintaining Your Progress	10
Phase 1: The release	10
Phase 2: Reboot	11
Phase 3: Reinstate	11
The Next Phase of Maintenance	12
BREAKFAST BOOSTERS	14
Energizing Morning Meals to Kickstart Your Day	14
Nutrient-Packed Smoothies and Shakes for Sustained Energy	16
WHOLESOME LUNCHES And SATISFYING SALADS	19
Flavorful and Filling Lunchtime Options	19
Fresh and Creative Salad Combinations to Keep You Satisfied	21
NOURISHING DINNERS	24
Delicious Dinners for the Whole Family to Enjoy	24
One-Pan Wonders: Easy and Healthy Dinner Solutions	26
GUILT- FREE SNACKS AND APPETIZERS	29
On-the-Go Snacks to Keep Cravings at Bay	29
Flavorful Appetizers for Social Gatherings and Parties	31

SWEET TREATS, GOLO-STYLE ... 34
  Smart Dessert Choices to Satisfy Your Sweet Tooth ... 34
  Baking with Balance: Healthier Dessert Alternatives ... 36
GOLO DIET ON SPECIAL OCCASIONS ... 38
  Celebratory Recipes without Compromising Your Progress ... 38
  Smart Strategies for Dining Out on the GOLO Diet ... 40
INCORPORATING EXERCISE INTO YOUR GOLO JOURNEY ... 42
  The Role of Physical Activity in Weight Loss ... 42
  Tailoring Exercise to Complement Your GOLO Diet Plan ... 44
MAINTAINING YOUR PROGRESS AND EMBRACING A HEALTHIER... ... 47
  Building Lasting Habits for Continued Success ... 47
  Overcoming Challenges and Staying Motivated on the GOLO Diet ... 50
FREQUENTLY ASKED QUESTIONS ABOUT THE GOLO DIET ... 53
  Addressing Common Concerns and Misconceptions ... 53
    The GOLO Diet: Is it a Fad? ... 53
    2. Does the GOLO diet necessitate calorie counting? ... 54
    3. Could Nutrient Deficiencies Occur Due to the GOLO Diet? ... 54
    4. Will the GOLO Diet Still Allow Me to Enjoy Carbohydrates? ... 54
    5. Can Anyone Follow the GOLO Diet? ... 54
    6. Will the GOLO Diet Cause Me to Lose Weight Quickly? ... 55
    7. Can I Follow the GOLO Diet Without Any Restrictions? ... 55
    8. Do Expensive Supplements Need to Be Taken with the GOLO Diet? ... 55
EXPERT INSIGHTS AND TIPS FOR OPTIMIZING YOUR GOLO EXPERIENCE ... 57
CONCLUSION: EMBRACE THE GOLO DIET FOR SUSTAINABLE WEIGHT... ... 60
  Recap of Key Takeaways ... 60
    Key Learnings: ... 60
SUCCESS STORIES ... 62
YOUR PATH TO A HEALTHIER AND HAPPIER YOU! ... 64

INTRODUCTION

Greetings and welcome to the "GOLO Diet Cookbook," your indispensable roadmap for a delicious and revolutionary path towards long-term weight loss and enhanced wellbeing.

We provide a selection of tasty, nutrient-dense meals that have been meticulously chosen to go along with the ground-breaking GOLO Diet in the pursuit of a healthy way of life.

The GOLO Diet is a science-based weight control strategy that goes beyond quick cures, not just another trend.

It emphasizes comprehending the complex interaction between insulin, metabolism, and weight loss while providing a balanced and all-encompassing approach to reaching your health objectives.

With this cookbook in your possession, you'll set out on a delicious culinary journey that complements the GOLO Diet's guiding principles.

We set the stage for your adventure in the first chapters. Learn everything there is to know about the GOLO Diet, its guiding principles, and how it differs from other dieting approaches.

Investigate the advantages it offers, including weight loss and promoting constant energy, mental clarity, and general vitality.

As you move closer to your weight loss objectives, we'll support you as you move through the GOLO Diet's many phases.

This cookbook is made to suit all levels of experience, whether you are new to the GOLO Diet or seeking to maximize your results.

The GOLO Diet's core principle of nourishing your body with the correct meals is where our recipes come into play.

With our invigorating morning meals and wonderful smoothies that give you the best start to your hectic day, breakfast will quickly become your favorite meal of the day.

With a variety of healthy choices and inventive salad combinations, lunches will be converted into enjoyable experiences that will leave you feeling filled and energized.

Our family-friendly supper options will tantalize your taste buds with delectable dishes, and our one-pan miracles will make meal preparation easier without sacrificing flavor or nutrition.

Since we know how important snacks and starters are to any diet, we have developed clever, guilt-free strategies to help you satisfy your desires.

And yes, desserts are acceptable. Enjoy our delectable snacks GOLO-style without stopping what you're doing.

Additionally, this cookbook explores how to handle special occasions and eat out while adhering to the GOLO Diet.

Celebrations don't have to be a time of sacrifice, but rather a chance to have fun without thinking twice.

We emphasize the importance of incorporating physical activity into your

GOLO journey to compliment your culinary accomplishments.

Learn how combining exercise with a healthy diet can improve your results and overall wellbeing.

We provide advice on how to sustain your progress, get beyond setbacks, and adopt a healthier way of life as you start down this revolutionary journey.

The "GOLO Diet Cookbook" is a plan for long-term change and a healthier, happier you; it is more than just a collection of dishes.

Therefore, let's go out on this fascinating journey together! For a happier, healthier future, embrace the flavors, embrace the balance, and embrace the GOLO Diet.

Make each meal a celebration of hydration and vitality as the first step in your personal change.

BOOK DESCRIPTION

The GOLO Diet Cookbook Unlocks the Key to Long-Term Weight Loss and Radiant Health

With the GOLO Diet Cookbook, learn a cutting-edge method for nourishing your body and reducing extra pounds.

This fascinating book, written by renowned nutritionist Dr. Olivia Wells, is filled with mouthwatering recipes, knowledgeable advice, and scientifically supported success strategies.

Say goodbye to restrictive diets and hello to a tasty, balanced meal that will boost your metabolism and normalize your blood sugar levels.

These nutrient-dense dishes range from invigorating breakfasts to delectable dinners the whole family will enjoy, keeping you nourished and inspired on your quest for wellbeing.

By incorporating the basic rules and principles for success, you may navigate eating out with ease and indulge in sensible dessert decisions without feeling guilty.

Learn how to build enduring habits, overcome obstacles, and maintain motivation for ongoing improvement.

Change your life by becoming a part of the GOLO Diet movement.

With the GOLO Diet Cookbook, you can begin your journey to a better, happier self right away.

INTRODUCTION TO THE GOLO DIET

Understanding the GOLO Diet: A Science-based Approach to Weight Loss

For a very long time, millions of people all around the world have struggled with their weight.

Numerous diets have appeared, promising quick fixes and miracle treatments, but they frequently turn out to be unsustainable or inefficient over time.

The GOLO Diet, in contrast, is a science-based strategy that focuses on the subtleties of the body's metabolism and insulin response in an effort to reveal the secrets of weight loss.

The GOLO Diet, at its foundation, goes beyond calorie tracking or imposing stringent limitations. Instead, it explores the intricate interactions between insulin, metabolism, and weight control.

Understanding this link is essential to understanding why some people may find it difficult to lose weight despite following a typical diet.

The hormone insulin, which is made by the pancreas, is essential for controlling blood sugar levels.

When we eat carbs, our bodies convert them to glucose, which raises blood sugar levels.

Insulin is then released by the pancreas to transport glucose into the cells, where it is utilised as a source of energy. Glucose that is in excess is stored as fat.

Many people can have an ongoing cycle of insulin resistance, which forces the body to create more insulin in order to keep blood sugar levels stable.

In turn, elevated insulin levels tell the body to store more fat, making it harder to lose weight.

This occurrence has the potential to start a vicious cycle that results in weight gain, increased insulin resistance, and harder weight loss.

The GOLO Diet aims to end this cycle by emphasizing three key pillars:

1. **Metabolic Health:** The GOLO Diet seeks to more successfully and sustainably support weight loss by treating insulin resistance and striving to improve metabolic health.

2. **Balanced Nutrition**: The GOLO Diet stresses balanced nutrition, integrating the proper proportion of proteins, carbs, and fats to regulate blood sugar levels and enhance metabolism, unlike fad diets that eliminate entire food groups.

3. **Nutritional Timing**: The GOLO Diet places a strong emphasis on the timing of our meals in order to maintain constant blood sugar levels throughout the day and prevent energy slumps and overeating.

The GOLO Diet's tailored approach is one of its defining qualities. Given that every person has a different physiology, the diet customizes its suggestions based on things like age, gender, amount of activity, and metabolism.

This tailored approach enables a more focused and long-lasting weight loss program.

The GOLO Diet is not a temporary solution, though. To support long-term success, it promotes the adoption of wholesome dietary practices and lifestyle adjustments.

The goal of the diet is to establish a sustainable route to a better and happier life by encouraging gradual and consistent weight loss.

It is crucial to approach your GOLO Diet adventure with patience and an open mind as you get started.

Knowing the science behind the diet will give you the power to make wise decisions and adopt a new eating style that nourishes your body and improves your health.

Keep in mind that the GOLO Diet is about more than just reducing weight; it's also about taking back control of your health and living a healthy, vibrant life.

So let's explore the guiding principles and advantages of this science-based weight loss strategy in further detail and see how the GOLO Diet can change your life.

Benefits of the GOLO Diet for Long-term Health and Well-being

There is much more to achieving a better and more satisfying life than merely losing weight quickly.

With its science-based approach to weight control, the GOLO Diet offers a plethora of advantages that go far beyond short-term health and general wellbeing.

Let's examine how the GOLO Diet might enhance your life in ways that go beyond reducing weight.

1. **Sustainable Weight Loss**: The GOLO Diet's focus on enhancing metabolic health and tackling insulin resistance paves the way for long-term weight loss.

The diet fosters healthy, long-lasting changes while avoiding the problems of yo-yo dieting by encouraging gradual and steady growth.

2. **Balanced Blood Sugar Levels**: The GOLO Diet helps maintain consistent blood sugar levels by carefully selecting meals that balance macronutrients and regulate portion sizes.

This helps with weight management as well as improving mood and supplying more energy throughout the day.

3. **Increased Energy and Vitality**: The GOLO Diet maintains sustained energy levels and lessens the chance of energy crashes after meals by optimizing insulin response and nutrient absorption.

The increased sense of wellbeing that results from this newfound vigour makes it simpler to maintain everyday activity and engagement.

4. **Improved Cardiovascular Health:** The GOLO Diet's emphasis on foods high in nutrients, like whole grains, lean meats, and healthy fats, may help to improve cardiovascular health.

The diet promotes heart health and lowers the chance of developing certain chronic illnesses by limiting consumption of refined carbs and harmful fats.

5. **Better Digestive Health:** Emphasizing the consumption of foods high in fiber and nutrients promotes good digestive health.

The general health of the digestive system can be enhanced by improved nutrition absorption, decreased bloating, and encouraged regular bowel movements in the gut.

6. **Improved Cognitive performance and Mental Clarity**: The GOLO Diet's stable blood sugar levels can help to increase cognitive performance and mental clarity.

Improved concentration, memory retention, and general cognitive performance can result from less energy swings.

7. **Reducing Inflammation**: Chronic diseases and other health problems, including inflammation, have been related to one another.

Inflammation can be reduced and a healthy internal environment can be promoted by the GOLO Diet's emphasis on complete, unprocessed foods and anti-inflammatory substances.

8. **Support for Hormonal Balance:** Improved metabolic health and balanced blood sugar levels can have a good impact on how hormones are regulated.

This can help women who suffer from illnesses like polycystic ovarian syndrome (PCOS) and can also help men and women with hormonal balance.

9. **Improved Sleep Quality**: The GOLO Diet's emphasis on balanced nutrition and food timing can have a good effect on sleep quality.

A more restful night's sleep can result from stable blood sugar levels throughout the day.

10. **Enhanced Longevity**: The GOLO Diet creates the conditions for enhanced longevity by encouraging healthy eating practices and lifestyle adjustments.

Long-term diet adherence can lead to a healthier, fuller life with a lower chance of aging-related health problems.

In conclusion, the GOLO Diet has several advantages that go well beyond weight loss.

The GOLO Diet equips people to take long-term control of their health by recognizing and addressing the underlying causes of weight management, such as insulin resistance and metabolic health.

Adopting the GOLO Diet is not simply a short-term dietary choice; it is a life-transforming option that will lead to a happier and more vibrant future with prolonged energy, increased mood, and overall better health.

GETTING STARTED WITH THE GOLO DIET

Essential Principles and Guidelines for Success

The GOLO Diet is a potent, scientifically supported method of weight management that aims to support long-term weight loss and general wellbeing.

Understanding and following the guiding concepts and rules that form the foundation of the GOLO Diet is key to maximizing your chances of success on this transforming journey.

The following guidelines will help you have a successful GOLO experience:

1. **Balance and Moderation:** The GOLO Diet places an emphasis on eating in a balanced way by including a variety of nutrient-dense meals from all of the major food groups.

To make sure you get the nutrients you need for good health, stay away from excessive limits and concentrate on moderation.

2. **Consider the timing of your meals** and snacks when consuming nutrients.

To balance blood sugar levels and minimize energy dumps, the GOLO Diet promotes regular meal schedules throughout the day. Try to eat frequently and at the right times for snacks.

3. **Portion Control**: Pay attention to portion sizes to prevent overeating and to maintain a balanced intake of calories.

Although the GOLO Diet does not include precise calorie counting, portion control is essential to weight loss and proper management of insulin response.

4. **Select whole Foods**: Whenever feasible, choose entire, unadulterated foods.

These consist of entire grains, lean proteins, lean veggies, fresh fruits, and healthy fats.

Avoid highly refined and processed foods, which are frequently high in harmful fats and added sugars.

5. **Watch Your Carbohydrate Intake**: The GOLO Diet relies heavily on carbohydrates, but it's important to pick the proper ones.

Reduce your diet of refined carbs and sugary meals while increasing your intake of complex carbohydrates like those found in whole grains and veggies.

6. **Hydration**: Throughout the day, drink enough water. Water is essential for overall health, and staying properly hydrated can assist your body's metabolic processes and help you avoid reaching for unhealthy snacks.

7. **Regular Exercise**: The GOLO Diet promotes including regular exercise in your daily routine. Exercise enhances overall wellbeing by accelerating metabolism, promoting cardiovascular health, and supplementing the diet.

To make fitness a sustainable part of your lifestyle, engage in activities you find enjoyable.

8. **Maintain Consistency**: The GOLO Diet requires consistency for success. Respect the guiding principles and refrain from regularly deviating from them.

The best outcomes will be obtained over time with dedication to the diet and lifestyle adjustments.

9. **Pay Attention to Your Body's Cues**: Listen to your body's signals of hunger and fullness. Instead of overeating out of habit or out of emotion, eat consciously and stop when you are full.

10. **Have Kindness and Patience with Yourself**: Changing your lifestyle and losing weight takes time and effort. Accept the path and practice self-compassion.

Celebrate modest victories and take lessons from failures. Keep in mind that progress, not perfection, is what drives lasting change.

11. **Seek Support**: Take into account asking for help from family, friends, or a group of people who are also on the GOLO Diet.

With others who share similar goals and struggles, you can get inspiration and accountability.

You'll position yourself for success on the GOLO Diet by adhering to these fundamental concepts and recommendations.

Celebrate the benefits it gives to your health and general well-being while embracing the process and the tasty and nourishing food.

The GOLO Diet is a radical lifestyle shift that opens the door to a healthier and happy you; it is not just a temporary diet.

GOLO Diet Phases: Transitioning and Maintaining Your Progress

The GOLO Diet is divided into various phases, each of which has a distinct goal for your road to wellness and weight loss.

For successful transitioning between these phases and maintaining your progress for long-term success, it is essential to comprehend these phases and their relevance.

Phase 1: The release

The GOLO Diet's Release phase is its first step, with an emphasis on helping you get started on your weight loss quest.

You'll rigorously adhere to the diet's instructions throughout this phase to balance blood sugar levels, lessen insulin resistance, and start burning fat.

Phase 1 of the diet is particularly crucial for implementing the concepts of balanced nutrition and portion control.

- Give whole, unprocessed foods top priority.

- Limit additional sweets and refined carbs.

- Consume three healthy meals and one snack each day.

- Drink water to stay hydrated.

- Add frequent physical activity.

Phase 2: Reboot

You will move on to the Reboot phase once you have achieved considerable progress in Phase 1.

Here, you'll introduce a more flexible strategy while maintaining the focus on healthy eating practices and long-term weight loss.

The Reboot phase is intended to sustain constant progress toward your objectives while further enhancing your metabolic health.

Key Recommendations:

- Keep eating mindfully and with balanced meals.

- Gradually add more items to the diet, including occasional pleasures in moderation.

- Modify portion sizes in accordance with your body's evolving needs.

- Continue your usual exercise regimen.

Phase 3: Reinstate

The Reinstate phase ushers in the shift to weight control and lifelong wellness.

You've now lost the weight you wanted to and are concentrating on keeping up your long-term progress.

The Reinstate phase places a strong emphasis on maintaining a healthy lifestyle, eating a balanced diet, and exercising regularly.

Key Recommendations:

- Adopt a more flexible approach to dietary selections, including a variety of nutrient-dense foods.

- Maintain a focus on healthy meals and portion control.

- Develop a mindful eating habit and pay attention to your body's signals of hunger and fullness.

- Find enjoyment in regular exercise and incorporate it into your daily routine.

- To maintain motivation, stay in touch with your support system or a group of like-minded people.

The Next Phase of Maintenance

The GOLO Diet's tenets start to permeate your lifestyle as soon as you pass the Reinstate phase.

The emphasis now switches to preserving your gains and making long-term, health-conscious decisions.

Keep in mind that maintaining a healthy weight requires continual effort, and sometimes adjustments are needed to accommodate physical and lifestyle changes.

It's important to be patient and kind to oneself at all times.

Progress may not always be linear when it comes to weight loss and lifestyle modifications.

Accept the journey, rejoice in your accomplishments, and take lessons from any failures.

Believe in the benefits of the GOLO Diet's science-based principles for your health and wellbeing.

You can confidently move through each stage of the GOLO Diet and sustain your progress toward living a healthier, happier, and more vibrant life by comprehending the diet's phases and diligently adhering to its principals.

The GOLO eating is a revolutionary and lasting method of nourishing your body and taking back control of your general well-being; it is not just a short-term eating regimen.

BREAKFAST BOOSTERS

Energizing Morning Meals to Kickstart Your Day

The start of your day, which establishes the tone for the hours to come, is in the morning.

An invigorating and nutrient-rich breakfast is crucial to kickingstart your metabolism, increasing your energy, and improving your general health.

We provide a selection of energizing morning meals in this section of the GOLO Diet Cookbook to help you get through the day.

1. **Nutrient-Rich Smoothies:** Smoothies are a great way to pack a range of nutrients into a single, tasty beverage. A protein- and fiber-rich smoothie made with a variety of leafy greens, fresh fruits, Greek yogurt, and chia seeds will keep you full and satisfied until your next meal.
2. **Filling Bowls of Oatmeal**: A hearty cup of warm oatmeal is a time-honored breakfast option that never fails. Add some sliced bananas, honey, and nuts or seeds for extra protein and good fats to it to increase its nutritional content.
3. **Pancakes Packed With Protein**: Who said pancakes couldn't be healthy? Using Greek yogurt, egg whites, and almond flour, make a protein-rich

pancake batter. For a breakfast that is both decadent and filling, top them with fresh berries and a dollop of Greek yogurt.
4. **Veggie Omelet**: For a delicious and veggie-rich omelet, whisk together eggs, spinach, bell peppers, and a dash of feta cheese. The vegetables offer a splash of color and taste, and the eggs are a fantastic source of protein and nutrients.
5. **Overnight Chia Pudding**: For a hassle-free morning, make this delicious breakfast the night before. Chia seeds should be combined with your preferred milk, some honey, and some vanilla extract. Wake morning to a creamy, nutrient-dense chia pudding that can be garnished with fresh fruit or nuts after letting it soak all night.
6. **Avocado Toast**: There is a solid reason why this dish has become a breakfast standard. Toast made from whole grains is topped with ripe avocado, sliced tomatoes, black pepper, and lime juice. This straightforward but filling combo offers fiber, good fats, and a rush of flavor.
7. **High-Protein Breakfast Burrito**: In a whole-wheat tortilla, roll together scrambled eggs, black beans, sautéed vegetables, and a dollop of salsa for a protein-rich breakfast burrito that will leave you feeling satiated and motivated all morning.
8. **Nut butter and banana sandwich**: Spread whole-grain bread with almond or peanut butter, then top with slices of banana. This delicious sandwich is a quick and stimulating breakfast alternative because it is full of fiber, potassium, and healthy fats.

The GOLO Diet is a gastronomic journey, and these stimulating morning dishes are just the beginning.

Every recipe has been meticulously created to offer the ideal ratio of nutrients to start your day off right and nourish your body.

Enjoy breakfast, fill your mornings with healthful deliciousness, and prepare yourself for a full and active day.

Nutrient-Packed Smoothies and Shakes for Sustained Energy

Smoothies and shakes are the ideal portable food options for giving your body prolonged energy and necessary minerals.

These delectable concoctions, which are brimming with vitamins, minerals, fiber, and protein, give a reviving pick-me-up during the afternoon slump or a refreshing and practical way to start your day.

We offer a delicious selection of nutrient-rich smoothies and shakes in this area of the GOLO Diet Cookbook that will make you feel energised and satiated.

1. **Green Power Smoothie**: Mix a cup of milk or a dairy-free substitute with a handful of spinach or kale, a frozen banana, a scoop of plant-based protein powder, a dollop of almond butter, and your choice of other fruits or vegetables.

You may power your day with a vivacious green smoothie that has been well blended and is high in iron, potassium, and protein.

2. **Berry Blast Shake**: Combine Greek yogurt, a splash of almond milk, and some flaxseeds or chia seeds with a variety of antioxidant-rich berries, including strawberries, blueberries, and raspberries.

This berrylicious shake will give you a flavorful kick and long-lasting energy to get you through the day.

3. **Tropical Paradise Smoothie**: With this delectable smoothie, travel to the tropics. A scoop of vanilla protein powder, some baby spinach, and frozen pineapple, mango, and coconut water are blended together.

The outcome is a vitamin and mineral-rich, moisturizing, and refreshing smoothie.

4. **Guilt-free Chocolate Banana Protein smoothie**: Satisfy your sweet taste while keeping on course with this smoothie. A ripe banana, a teaspoon of cocoa powder, a scoop of chocolate protein powder, and your preferred milk or milk substitute should all be blended together.

It is a filling, nutrient-rich treat that won't interfere with your efforts to improve your health.

5. **Almond Butter and Date Smoothie**: This creamy smoothie combines the richness of almond butter with the dates' inherent sweetness.

Almond milk, pitted dates, a scoop of vanilla protein powder, and almond butter should all be combined.

The outcome is a delicious smoothie that is high in protein and will satisfy hunger.

6. **Coffee and Oat Smoothie**: Try this coffee-infused smoothie for an extra morning boost. Your preferred coffee should be brewed, let to cool, and then blended with oats, a banana, protein powder, and a little almond milk.

For coffee fans who desire a nutritional boost, this smoothie is ideal.

7. **Peanut Butter and Jelly Shake**: Enjoy a healthier version of your favorite childhood treats. Greek yogurt, a scoop of peanut butter, a few drops of honey, and frozen mixed berries should all be blended together.

The end result is a protein- and nutrient-rich shake that is nostalgic but healthy.

8. **An energizing green tea smoothie** can be made by brewing some green tea, letting it cool, and then blending it with some frozen pineapple, cucumber, spinach, and protein powder.

This green tea smoothie gives you prolonged energy and a cooling punch of antioxidants.

These nutrient-dense shakes and smoothies are adaptable, enabling you to tailor them to your taste and dietary requirements.

These delectable concoctions will keep you invigorated and nourished throughout the day, whether you're searching for a quick breakfast choice, a post-workout refill, or a mid-afternoon energy boost.

Therefore, grab your blender and get ready to sip your way to long-lasting energy and vigor on the GOLO Diet!

WHOLESOME LUNCHES And SATISFYING SALADS

Flavorful and Filling Lunchtime Options

The opportunity to recharge your body with a filling and substantial meal at lunch will keep you alert and focused for the remainder of the day.

We offer an exquisite variety of flavorful and substantial lunch alternatives in this chapter of the GOLO Diet Cookbook that highlight a fusion of ingredients, textures, and global inspirations.

These lunchtime alternatives, which range from filling salads to healthy bowls and cozy wraps, will please your palate and keep you full until your next meal.

1. **Quinoa salad with Kalamata olives, cucumber, cherry tomatoes, feta cheese, and lemon vinaigrette**. Combine cooked quinoa with these ingredients.

This Mediterranean-inspired salad is a blast of flavors and textures that will leave you feeling satiated and nourished. It is garnished with a sprinkle of fresh herbs like mint and parsley.

2. **Chicken Avocado Wrap**: For a filling and protein-dense lunch option, wrap grilled chicken, avocado slices, mixed greens, and a dab of hummus in a whole-grain tortilla.

For a quick and portable lunch, this wrap offers a delicious combination of creamy avocado and flavorful chicken.

3. **Thai Peanut Noodle Bowl**: Combine cooked rice noodles with bell peppers, edamame, carrots, and a spicy peanut sauce.

For an unusual and full noodle bowl that satisfies your demands for both salty and nutty flavors, garnish with chopped cilantro and crushed peanuts.

4. **Grilled Vegetable Panini**: Place fresh mozzarella, grilled bell peppers, zucchini, eggplant, and eggplant between slices of whole-grain bread.

Paninis should be toasted until the cheese melts and the bread becomes crunchy. You'll want to keep eating this delectable sandwich because of the variety of flavors and textures it offers.

5. **Lentil and Roasted Vegetable Salad**: Roast a variety of seasonal vegetables, including red onions, sweet potatoes, and Brussels sprouts.

Combine the cooked lentils with the roasted vegetables and a tart balsamic vinaigrette.

This filling salad is a powerhouse of nutrition and plant-based protein.

6. **Sushi Inspired Brown Rice Bowl**: Add sliced avocado, cucumber, pickled ginger, imitation crab, or cooked shrimp to a bed of brown rice.

Pour over a soy sauce and sesame oil dressing for a healthful and umami-filled deconstructed sushi dish.

7. **Caprese Stuffed Pita**: Stuff fresh mozzarella, cherry tomatoes, and basil leaves into a whole-grain pita. For a tasty, quick-to-assemble Caprese-inspired lunch alternative, drizzle with balsamic glaze.

8. **Mexican quinoa bowl**: top cooked quinoa with salsa, roasted corn, black beans, and chopped avocado. Finish with a dollop of sour cream or Greek yogurt for a spicy, protein-rich bowl with a touch of Mexican flavor.

These scrumptious and substantial lunch alternatives offer the ideal ratio of necessary vitamins, flavors, and textures to keep you full and energized all day.

These healthy lunch options are a welcome addition to your GOLO Diet journey, whether you choose to eat them at home, pack them for work, or share them with loved ones.

So reward yourself with a satisfying and mouthwatering lunch and enjoy the pleasure of fueling your body with a range of fresh and healthy products!

Fresh and Creative Salad Combinations to Keep You Satisfied

When using fresh vegetables in abundance and being creative, salads are everything from dull.

We provide a variety of delicious salad combinations that will excite your taste buds and keep you feeling completely satiated in this section of the GOLO Diet Cookbook.

These salads offer an exquisite blend of nutrition and flavor sensations while celebrating brilliant colors, varied textures, and distinctive flavor profiles.

1. **Grilled Peach and Arugula Salad**: Toss ripe peaches with peppery arugula, crumbled goat cheese, and toasted almonds after grilling them until they are caramelized and smokey.

For a fulfilling and stylish sweet and savory salad, drizzle with balsamic glaze.

2. **Roasted Beet and Goat Cheese Salad**: Toss roasted beets with mixed greens, candied walnuts, and creamy goat cheese until they are soft and sweet.

For a salad that is earthy, deep, and totally wonderful, dress with a mild vinaigrette.

3. **Sesame Ginger Salad with an Asian Influence**:
   Combine mixed greens, diced bell peppers, cucumber, and carrots that have been shredded.

Add grilled chicken or tofu to the plate, then sprinkle on the tangy sesame ginger dressing.

This cooling salad features a tasteful fusion of Asian-inspired flavors and textures.

4. **Southwest Black Bean Salad**: Bring together black beans, corn, cherry tomatoes, cubed avocado, and chopped cilantro.

A robust, zesty salad with a Southwestern flair that is ideal for a satisfying lunch or light dinner can be dressed with a cumin-lime dressing.

5. **Mediterranean Watermelon Feta Salad**: Combine pieces of sweet, juicy watermelon with Kalamata olives, crumbled feta cheese, and fresh mint leaves.

For a breezy and cool salad that is a blast of sweet and savory delight, add a sprinkle of black pepper and a drizzle of olive oil.

6. **Orange and pomegranate-seed quinoa salad**: Combine cooked quinoa with finely chopped pistachios, fresh mint, and orange segments.

For a vibrant, nutrient-rich salad that is acidic and crunchy, dress with a lemon vinaigrette.

7. **Baby spinach, strawberry, and goat cheese salad**: Combine baby spinach, strawberry slices, goat cheese crumbles, and candied pecans. A balsamic reduction should be drizzled on top for a sweet and sour salad that showcases seasonal ingredients.

8. **Tex-Mex Taco Salad**: Top mixed greens with black beans, chopped tomatoes, shredded cheddar cheese, and crumbled tortilla chips. You can also use seasoned mince beef or turkey.

For a Tex-Mex-inspired salad that is a filling and healthy supper, top with a dollop of Greek yogurt or salsa.

The countless options that salads can provide are demonstrated by these vibrant and inventive salad combinations.

Enjoy the abundance of flavorful fresh ingredients available, and use your creativity to make unique salads by combining different elements.

These salads demonstrate that consuming wholesome foods doesn't require giving up flavor or satisfaction.

So start your trip on the GOLO Diet with a gastronomic adventure and discover the thrill of colorful, inventive salads that will keep you satiated.

NOURISHING DINNERS

Delicious Dinners for the Whole Family to Enjoy

Dinnertime gatherings with loved ones are treasured occasions full of joy, affection, and, of course, delicious meals.

The GOLO Diet Cookbook presents a variety of delicious dishes that the whole family will enjoy in this part.

These recipes range from comforting classics to those with global influences and are created to be tasty, wholesome, and family-friendly.

1. **Baked Parmesan Chicken**: Toss whole-grain breadcrumbs, grated Parmesan cheese, and Italian herbs together to coat chicken breasts.

For a filling and healthy dinner, bake the chicken until it is golden and crispy, then serve it with roasted vegetables on the side or a crisp green salad.

2. **Veggie-Packed Turkey Meatballs**: Mix shredded zucchini, carrots, and onions with lean ground turkey. Meatballs should be formed, then baked until fully cooked.

Serve this nutritious and kid-friendly variation of a traditional favorite with whole-grain spaghetti and marinara sauce.

3. **Quinoa-Stuffed Bell Peppers**: Stuff cooked quinoa, black beans, diced tomatoes, and spices into bell peppers to add flavor.

Bake the filling in the oven until it is thoroughly cooked and the peppers are soft. Add fresh cilantro and grated cheese for a colorful and nutrient-rich dinner alternative.

4. **Beef and Broccoli Stir-Fry**: Add strips of lean beef to a saucy sauce composed with low-sodium soy sauce, garlic, and ginger, along with broccoli florets, sliced bell peppers, and other vegetables.

For a simple and savory dinner that is guaranteed to be a favorite, serve over brown rice or cauliflower rice.

5. **Pesto Pasta with Grilled Shrimp**: Combine whole-grain pasta with grilled shrimp and homemade or store-bought pesto sauce.

For more color and minerals, mix with spinach and cherry tomatoes. The flavors and textures of this spaghetti dish are a lovely blend of seasonal ingredients.

6. **Sandwiches with BBQ pulled chicken**: Slow-cook chicken breasts in a tangy, smokey BBQ sauce until they are fork-tender.

For a family-pleasing dinner, shred the chicken and serve it on whole-grain buns with a side of coleslaw or a straightforward green salad.

7. **Vegetable and Chickpea Curry**: Combine a variety of aromatic spices, coconut milk, and a rainbow of colorful veggies to make a tasty vegetable and chickpea curry.

Serve over quinoa or brown rice for a filling and healthy dinner alternative.

8. **Margherita Pizza**: Make your own whole grain pizza dough and cover it with tomato sauce, sliced fresh mozzarella, and fresh basil.

Bake the pie until the crust is golden and the cheese is bubbling. For a crowd-pleasing dinner that's ideal for family pizza night, make this traditional Margherita pizza.

With these delectable dinners, the whole family will enjoy eating together because they are created to appeal to both adults and kids.

Enjoy these healthy and delicious meals and seize the chance to make lifelong memories at the dinner table.

These GOLO Diet family-friendly dinners, which emphasize using fresh ingredients and a variety of flavors, are guaranteed to become cherished favorites that bring everyone together for satisfying and enjoyable evenings.

One-Pan Wonders: Easy and Healthy Dinner Solutions

Dinner preparation doesn't have to be difficult or time-consuming. Discover the world of one-pan miracles, where wholesome meals may be prepared quickly and easily.

We offer a selection of quick and wholesome meal ideas that only call for one pan or skillet in this section of the GOLO Diet Cookbook.

Even the busiest households will find it easy to make dinner with these dishes, which range from delicious sheet pan meals to filling stir-fries.

1. **Salmon and Veggies in a Sheet Pan with Lemon and Herbs**: Arrange salmon fillets on a sheet pan and surround them with a vibrant assortment of in-season veggies, such as asparagus, cherry tomatoes, and baby potatoes.

drizzle with a concoction of fresh herbs, lemon juice, and olive oil. Bake the salmon until it's perfectly done and the vegetables are crisp-tender.

This one-pan marvel provides a filling and healthy supper all at once.

2. **One-Pot Chicken and Brown Rice**: In a big skillet, brown rice, diced veggies, and chicken stock are added after the chicken pieces have been cooked until browned.

Cook the rice and combine the spices in a simmering pot. This one-pot recipe is a filling and healthy dinner choice that the whole family will love.

3. **Veggie-Packed Shrimp Stir-Fry**: Stir-fry shrimp with a variety of vibrant veggies, including bell peppers, broccoli, and snap peas, in a wok or sizable pan. Add flavor with a low-sodium soy sauce, garlic, and ginger stir-fry sauce.

For a quick and filling dinner, serve over whole-grain noodles or cauliflower rice.

4. **Mexican quinoa in a single pan**:
   In a big skillet, cook ground beef or turkey with onions and bell peppers. Mix in the black beans, spices, diced tomatoes, and cooked quinoa. Add some cheese shavings on top, then let it melt.

This quick and easy dish with Mexican influences is a filling and nutrient-rich dinner.

5. **Lemon Garlic Herb Chicken and Potatoes**: In a skillet, brown chicken thighs with fresh herbs, garlic, and a blend of lemon juice. Potatoes should be added

and cooked with the chicken until fork-tender and flavorful.

The combination of delicate chicken and roasted potatoes in this one-pan marvel is delicious.

6. **One-Pan Pesto Chicken and Veggies**: Drizzle chicken breasts with pesto sauce and arrange them on a sheet pan with a variety of veggies, such as bell peppers, zucchini, and cherry tomatoes.

Roast the vegetables and chicken until they are both thoroughly done.

This quick meal option is flavored with fresh herbs and healthy ingredients.

7. **Teriyaki Tofu and Broccoli Skillet**: Stir-fry broccoli florets with tofu cubes in a skillet with a homemade teriyaki sauce made from low-sodium soy sauce, honey, ginger, and garlic.

For a filling, plant-based dinner that is rich in protein and nutrients, serve over brown rice.

These one-pan marvels are living proof that healthy and exquisite meals can be prepared quickly and without stress.

These dishes use straightforward, healthy ingredients and offer a range of flavors and textures to keep your taste buds happy and your dinner routine interesting.

Embrace the ease and simplicity of these quick and nutritious dinner ideas for the GOLO Diet, and you'll spend less time cooking while still sharing delicious and nourishing meals with your family.

GUILT- FREE SNACKS AND APPETIZERS

On-the-Go Snacks to Keep Cravings at Bay

Having quick and nourishing snacks on hand is crucial to fend off cravings and preserve energy when hunger strikes in between meals or while you're on the go.

We offer a variety of delicious and filling on-the-go snacks in this chapter of the GOLO Diet Cookbook.

These travel-friendly selections are ideal for crammed schedules, long drives, or whenever you need a fast pick-me-up.

1. **Trail Mix**: Mix a variety of raw nuts, seeds, and dried fruits to make your own trail mix.

The delicious combination of almonds, walnuts, pumpkin seeds, and dried cranberries is high in antioxidants and good fats.

2. **Veggie Sticks and Hummus**: Put bell pepper strips, thin slices of cucumber, and baby carrots in a little container.

The result will be a crispy, nutrient-rich snack that is ideal for dipping when combined with a portion of hummus.

3. **Greek Yogurt Parfait**: Arrange Greek yogurt, fresh fruit, and a dash of granola or nuts in a travel-friendly container.

Your appetites for sweets will be satisfied by this protein-rich parfait.

4. **Rice Cakes with Nut Butter**: Rice cakes with almond or peanut butter are a fast, crispy snack that is a rich source of protein and beneficial fats.

5. **Cheese and Whole-Grain Crackers**: For a flavorful and filling snack that's high in calcium and fiber, combine a few slices of your favorite cheese with whole-grain crackers.

6. **Energy Bites**: Make your own energy bites by mixing honey, nut butter, rolled oats, and optional ingredients like chia seeds, dried fruit, or dark chocolate chips.

Make bite-sized balls out of them for a quick and invigorating snack.

7. **Hard-Boiled Eggs**: For a portable, protein-rich snack, prepare hard-boiled eggs in advance and store them in the refrigerator.

8. **Fresh fruit**: Fruits that don't require much preparation and are high in vitamins and fiber include apples, bananas, and clementines.

9. **Seaweed Snacks**: Crispy roasted seaweed sheets satisfy your craving for a crunchy snack with a low-calorie and tasty solution.

10. **Dark Chocolate**: A tiny piece of dark chocolate with at least 70% cocoa content will satisfy a sweet tooth while also supplying antioxidants and mood-enhancing elements.

Keep in mind to stay hydrated by having a water bottle with you since hunger and thirst might occasionally be confused.

Even on hectic days, you can make healthier decisions and sate cravings by keeping these portable snacks on hand.

On the GOLO Diet, embrace the portability and delectability of these portable snacks and fill your body with nutritional foods that promote your general wellbeing.

Flavorful Appetizers for Social Gatherings and Parties

Without a delicious selection of appetizers that tempt the taste buds and set the tone for the occasion, a successful social gathering or party is left wanting.

The tasty and popular appetizers we offer in this area of the GOLO Diet Cookbook are sure to impress and leave your visitors begging for more.

These appetizers are the ideal way to start off any celebration with elegance and taste, from savory snacks to zesty dips.

1. **Caprese Skewers**: Thread basil leaves, cherry tomatoes, and fresh mozzarella balls onto tiny skewers. For a vibrant and energizing snack that honors the traditional Caprese flavors, drizzle with balsamic glaze.

2. **Spinach and Artichoke Dip**: Make a rich, creamy spinach and artichoke dip and serve it with whole-wheat pita chips or sliced vegetables. This cozy, decadent dip is a perennial favorite at gatherings.

3. **Stuffed small Peppers**: Stuff halved small peppers with a cream cheese

mixture that includes diced sun-dried tomatoes, minced herbs, and. Roast the peppers until they are soft and the filling is delicious and creamy.

4. **Smoked Salmon Cucumber Bites**: Place smoked salmon on cucumber slices and top with Greek yogurt or cream cheese and fresh dill. For a sophisticated event, these refined and light snacks are ideal.

5. **Chicken Satay Skewers:** Grill or bake chicken strips until fully cooked after marinating them in a fragrant satay sauce. For a delectable appetizer that is brimming with Asian flavors, serve with a peanut dipping sauce.

6. **Zucchini Fritters**: Finely grate the zucchini and combine it with the eggs, almond flour, and minced herbs. Create fritters out of the mixture, then pan-fry them till crisp and golden. These nutrient-dense fritters make a great and healthy appetizer.

7. **Mediterranean Hummus tray**: Arrange different types of hummus, olives, cherry tomatoes, cucumber slices, and whole-grain pita bread on a colorful tray. This spread with Mediterranean influences is a delicious way to display a range of tastes and textures.

8. **Cherry Tomatoes with Guacamole Stuffed Insides**: Scoop out the insides of cherry tomatoes and stuff them with your own guacamole. For a flavorful and attractive appetizer, garnish with fresh cilantro or chili powder.

9. **Vegetable Spring Rolls with Dipping Sauce**: In rice paper, encase a combination of fresh veggies, rice noodles, and herbs. For a tasty and light snack, serve the spring rolls with a peanut dipping sauce.

10. **Shrimp Cocktail**: Arrange a dish of tart cocktail sauce around chilled shrimp. Add lemon wedges and fresh parsley for a sophisticated and time-tested starter that will dazzle.

GUILT- FREE SNACKS AND APPETIZERS

The secret to organizing a memorable and fun party or social event is these tasty appetizers.

These crowd-pleasing appetizers are sure to please visitors of all ages, whether it's a casual gathering or a major celebration.

So, on the GOLO Diet, embrace the culinary experience and enjoy the pleasure of sharing delicious appetizers that enhance the ambiance and make every meeting a special occasion.

SWEET TREATS, GOLO-STYLE

Smart Dessert Choices to Satisfy Your Sweet Tooth

Your attempts to eat healthily need not be derailed by indulging in a sweet treat.

In this chapter of the GOLO Diet Cookbook, we provide a variety of sensible dessert options that will sate your sweet desire while keeping adhering to the GOLO Diet's core values.

These desserts are delicious and guilt-free ways to end a meal because they are crafted with healthy ingredients and have less added sugar.

1. **Fruit Salad with Honey-Lime Dressing**: Combine seasonal fruits including berries, melons, and citrus to make a vibrant fruit salad. Dress with a simple honey, lime, and a touch of cinnamon dressing. This cool treat is a celebration of vitamins and natural sweetness.

2. **Greek Yogurt Parfait with Berries**: To add some crunch, top the parfait with a layer of Greek yogurt and fresh berries. This parfait is a filling meal that will satisfy your want for something sweet. It is high in protein.

3. **Chia Seed Pudding with Fresh Fruit**: Chia seeds are soaked in either almond

or coconut milk to make chia seed pudding. For a thick and creamy dessert, top with sliced fresh fruit like mango, kiwi, or berries.

4. **Melted dark chocolate with at least 70% cocoa** content should be dipped into fresh strawberries. Enjoy a sweet and healthy dessert that is rich in antioxidants once the chocolate has had time to set.

5. **Baked apples with cinnamon**: Cut apples in half and stuff each half with a mixture of cinnamon, chopped almonds, and honey. Bake the apples until they are soft and fragrant. This soothing, healthy treat is a warm, spicy dessert.

6. Make **frozen banana** pops by placing popsicle sticks inside of peeled bananas and freezing them until solid. You can also put chopped almonds or coconut flakes on top after dipping the frozen bananas in melted dark chocolate. The fun and guilt-free way to enjoy a frozen treat is with these frozen banana pops.

7. **Coconut Mango Rice Pudding**: Stir together coconut milk, sliced mango, and brown rice until smooth and aromatic. Put a little honey or maple syrup over it to make it sweeter. Rice pudding with a tropical flair is a delicious and creamy delicacy.

8. **Almond Butter Date Bites**: In a food processor, mix almond butter, pitted dates, and a tiny bit of vanilla essence until a sticky dough forms. Refrigerate after forming the mixture into bite-sized balls. For a quick sweet fix, try these dessert energy bites, which are sweet and filling.

These shrewd dessert selections demonstrate that you can indulge in sweetness without jeopardizing your wellbeing.

On the GOLO Diet, embrace the goodness of healthy ingredients and natural flavors, and savor the delight of dessert.

You may indulge your sweet appetite while also promoting your general wellbeing and upholding a balanced and sustainable approach to healthy eating by making thoughtful and wholesome decisions.

Baking with Balance: Healthier Dessert Alternatives

It's possible to make delectable desserts that are both rich and healthful through baking, which may be a great and calming activity.

We offer a variety of baking recipes in this section of the GOLO Diet Cookbook that emphasize balance, use wholesome foods, and cut back on added sugars and bad fats.

With these treats, you may still adhere to the GOLO Diet's guiding principles while also experiencing the joy of baking.

1. **Whole Wheat Banana Bread**: Replace the refined flour in your favorite banana bread recipe with whole wheat flour. For natural sweetness and flavor, incorporate ripe bananas, a small amount of honey or maple syrup, and a dash of cinnamon.

2. **Oatmeal Raisin Cookies**: To make these delightful cookies, combine rolled oats, raisins, and a tiny bit of honey or date paste. These cookies are a filling treat because to the fiber and texture provided by the oats.

3. **Almond flour brownies**: Use almond flour in place of regular flour while making brownies. For a rich and fudgy treat, combine cocoa powder, dark chocolate chips, and a tiny quantity of coconut sugar or another natural sweetener of your choice.

4. **Coconut Flour Lemon Bars**: Create lemon bars with a coconut oil and flour

crust. For a tart flavor, add fresh lemon juice and zest. To add sweetness, stir in a little honey or stevia.

5. **Protein-Packed Muffins**: To make protein-packed muffins, combine Greek yogurt, a variety of fresh or frozen berries, and protein powder. These muffins are a portable, nutrient-rich alternative for a filling dessert or a speedy snack.

6. **Flourless Peanut Butter Cookies**: Combine natural peanut butter, an egg, and a little honey or maple syrup in a bowl and whisk to combine. Create little dough balls, then flatten each one with a fork. Enjoy these gluten-free, protein-packed cookies after baking until they are golden.

7. **Chia Seed Chocolate Pudding**: Combine chia seeds, almond milk, and a natural sweetener with unsweetened chocolate powder. Refrigerate the mixture until it thickens into a rich and wholesome chocolate pudding.

8. **Carrot Zucchini Bread:** To add moisture and nutrition to your bread recipe, use finely chopped carrots and zucchini. Warming spices like cinnamon and nutmeg can be used after you've added a tiny amount of honey or maple syrup to sweeten.

When baking, it's important to choose healthful ingredients, limit added sugars, and whenever possible, use nutrient-dense products.

With these healthier dessert options, you may continue to follow the GOLO Diet's guidelines while still getting the same pleasure from creating and indulging in sweet sweets.

So, embrace dessert making creativity while keeping your health in mind, and enjoy the satisfaction of enjoying healthier desserts that nourish and satisfy you.

GOLO DIET ON SPECIAL OCCASIONS

Celebratory Recipes without Compromising Your Progress

You shouldn't have to sacrifice your progress on the GOLO Diet in order to enjoy celebrations and special occasions.

We offer a selection of festive meals that are tasty and considerate of your health objectives in this area of the GOLO Diet Cookbook.

These dishes use healthy ingredients and clever replacements to fuel your body while letting you partake in the festivities.

1. **Herb Grilled Salmon**: Combine olive oil, lemon juice, garlic, and your preferred herbs to marinate fresh salmon. Serve grilled food that has been cooked to perfection with roasted veggies on the side or a crisp salad. This festive dish is both classy and wholesome.

2. **Quinoa Stuffed Bell Peppers**: Fill vibrant bell peppers with cooked quinoa, lean mince beef or turkey, diced tomatoes, and a mixture of flavorful spices. Bake the filling in the oven until it is flavorful and gratifying and the peppers are soft.

3. **Cauliflower Rice Sushi Rolls**: Create a sushi roll by combining cauliflower

rice, sliced avocado, cucumber, and imitation crab or cooked shrimp. Serve with wasabi, low-sodium soy sauce, and pickled ginger for a tasty and light sushi celebration.

4. **Baked Garlic Herb Chicken**: Drizzle a little olive oil, fresh herbs, and garlic over chicken thighs or breasts. Bake the chicken until it is tender and flavorful. Steamed veggies should be served as a side dish for a straightforward yet tasty festive feast.

5. **Vegetable Quiche with Whole Grain Crust**: Create a quiche that is filled with veggies by using a whole-grain crust, eggs, milk or a dairy-free substitute, and a variety of vibrant vegetables. It's the ideal dish for brunch or special occasions.

6. **Portobello Mushroom Burger**: Make burger patties out of grilled or baked Portobello mushroom caps that have been baked or grilled until they are fork-tender. Add your preferred condiments, such as lettuce, tomatoes, and avocado. Serve with lettuce wraps or whole-grain buns for a delicious and gratifying celebration.

7. **Grilled Vegetable Platter**: Cook a variety of seasonal vegetables, including asparagus, bell peppers, zucchini, and eggplant. For a delicious and healthy celebration, serve them with a tart hummus or balsamic glaze.

8. **Fruit Sorbet Parfait**: For a light and energizing dessert option, layer fruit sorbet with fresh berries and a dollop of Greek yogurt. This parfait is a refreshing and tasty way to cap off a festive lunch.

These festive recipes show that it's possible to follow the GOLO Diet and still partake in delectable meals.

You can prepare celebration meals that energize your body and make special occasions more enjoyable by putting a focus on full, nutrient-dense ingredients and making conscious decisions.

Therefore, rejoice in the knowledge that you can savor delicious sensations without jeopardizing your advancement toward health and well-being.

Smart Strategies for Dining Out on the GOLO Diet

Going out to eat can be difficult while you're on the GOLO Diet, but with some clever tactics, you can still enjoy yourself while maintaining your health objectives.

Here are some suggestions to assist you in making thoughtful decisions and keeping up your progress when dining out:

1. **Make a plan**: If at all feasible, research the menu of the restaurant online before visiting. By doing this, you may weigh your options and make a wise decision in advance rather than acting on the spur of the moment.

2. **Select Restaurants with Healthier Options**: Select eateries with a range of wholesome and fresh options, such as those that have an emphasis on salads, grilled proteins, and whole grains. Nowadays, a lot of restaurants provide healthier menu options or designate certain dishes as "light" or "healthy."

3. **Put an emphasis on Lean Proteins**: Look for dishes that include grilled lean meats like chicken, fish, or tofu. These choices are filling and help your body get the nutrition it needs.

4. **Be Aware of Portion Sizes**: Portion sizes at restaurants can differ from what you might regularly consume at home. Think about splitting an entree with a companion or ordering a to-go box to save half the meal for later.

5. **Keep an eye out for Hidden Sugars and Fats**: Sauces, dressings, and condiments may include extra sugars and bad fats. To limit how much you use of the dressings and sauces, request them on the side.

6. **Customization Is Important**: Don't be hesitant to request changes to accommodate your dietary preferences. For instance, you can ask for a salad without croutons or steamed vegetables rather than fries.

7. **Fill Up on veggies**: Opt for dishes that are full of veggies and concentrate on giving your food color and nutrients.

8. **Hydrate Smartly**: Choose water or unsweetened drinks over sugary sodas or mixed drinks. Your general health depends on staying hydrated, which can also aid in hunger control.

9. **Skip the Bread Basket**: To avoid consuming extra calories before your dinner, think twice if the restaurant offers you a bread basket.

10. **Be Aware of Desserts**: If you desire dessert, think about sharing it with others or choosing something healthy, such sorbet or fresh fruit.

Remember that dining out should be fun, and with these helpful tips, you may confidently peruse restaurant menus while adhering to the GOLO Diet.

You can enjoy the pleasures of restaurant food without jeopardizing your progress toward a healthier and more balanced lifestyle by making thoughtful decisions and balancing your meals with nutritious ingredients.

INCORPORATING EXERCISE INTO YOUR GOLO JOURNEY

The Role of Physical Activity in Weight Loss

The ability to lose weight and improve general health depends on physical activity.

Regular exercise can considerably help achieve and maintain a healthy body weight when accompanied with a balanced diet.

Here are some important ways that exercise helps people lose weight:

1. **Caloric Expenditure**: Physical activity, including strength training, aerobic exercise, and even regular tasks like walking or gardening, burns calories.

A calorie deficit is produced when you burn more calories than you take in, which over time causes you to lose weight.

2. **Increases Metabolism**: Your metabolic rate, or the number of calories your body burns while at rest, can be raised by regular physical exercise.

This implies that you'll burn more calories even when you're not exercising, aiding weight loss attempts.

3. **Preserves Lean Muscle Mass**: When shedding pounds, there is a chance that both muscle and fat will be lost.

Lean muscle mass needs to be preserved in order to maintain a healthy metabolism and body composition, which is made possible by strength training exercises.

4. **Increases Insulin Sensitivity**: By increasing insulin sensitivity, regular exercise helps your body utilise glucose more efficiently.

This can assist in controlling blood sugar levels and preventing the storage of extra glucose as fat.

5. **Suppresses Appetite**: Exercise has the potential to minimize hunger pangs and possibly prevent overeating by helping to suppress appetite hormones.

6. **Exercise releases endorphins**, which are naturally uplifting chemicals. This improves mental wellbeing.

This can lead to healthier eating patterns and improved weight management by lowering stress and emotional eating.

7. **boosts Energy Expenditure**: Exercising at a moderate to severe intensity boosts calorie expenditure during the exercise session and may cause an afterburn effect, where your body continues to burn calories after the exercise session.

8. **Encourages Long-Term Weight Maintenance**: Maintaining weight reduction and avoiding weight gain require incorporating regular physical exercise into your routine.

It promotes overall wellbeing and aids in the development of healthy behaviors.

It's important to remember that while exercise helps people lose weight, it is only one part of a comprehensive strategy for leading a healthy lifestyle.

For effective weight loss and maintenance, a balanced diet that includes nutrient-dense meals and sensible portion control is essential.

It's imperative to speak with a healthcare provider before beginning any workout regimen, especially if you have any current medical ailments or worries.

They can assist in creating an appropriate workout regimen that fits your demands for both general health and weight loss.

A good diet and regular exercise are a potent combination for attaining and maintaining weight loss while enhancing general health and wellbeing.

Tailoring Exercise to Complement Your GOLO Diet Plan

Regular exercise can improve your outcomes and assist your general health and well-being as you start your GOLO Diet journey.

You can accomplish your weight reduction and fitness objectives more quickly and efficiently by designing your workout program to work in conjunction with your GOLO Diet plan.

Here are some suggestions for adjusting your exercise routine so that it complements your diet:

1. **Speak with a Healthcare expert**: It's important to speak with a healthcare expert before beginning any fitness program, especially if you have any current medical ailments or concerns.

They may offer tailored advice and make sure that your workout program fits your particular requirements and objectives.

2. **Pick Activities You Enjoy**: Pick physical activities and exercises that you actually enjoy. Include activities you enjoy in your fitness routine, whether they be dancing, swimming, hiking, or cycling.

This will help you stay motivated and dedicated to your workout program.

3. **Balance Cardio and Strength Training**: Include a combination of cardio workouts in your program, such as jogging, cycling, or walking, as well as strength training, such as utilizing weights or bodyweight exercises.

Strength training keeps muscle mass and speeds metabolism while aerobic exercises assist burn calories and enhance cardiovascular health.

4. **Plan Regular Workouts**: Allocate specific time each day or several times per week for exercising. To make progress and profit from exercise, consistency is essential.

5. **Warm-Up and Cool-Down**: Make sure to warm up before working out to get your body ready, and cool down afterwards to gradually drop your heart rate and avoid sore muscles.

6. **High-Intensity Interval Training (HIIT)**: Take into account including HIIT into your daily exercise regimen. HIIT entails quick bursts of intensive exercise interspersed with moments of rest.

It might be a quick approach to lose weight and get more fit.

7. **Listen to Your Body**: Pay close attention to how exercise affects your body. It's acceptable to reduce the intensity or take rest days if you're feeling tired or painful so that your body can heal.

8. **Stay Hydrated**: To stay hydrated, drink plenty of water before, during, and after exercise, especially if you work out hard or work out outside in the heat.

9. **Maintain Flexibility**: Since life is unpredictable, there may be days when your workout schedule is interfered with. Be adaptable and ready to change your workout routine as necessary.

10. **Celebrate Your Progress**: No matter how tiny, celebrate your successes and advancements. You may increase your motivation and maintain your adherence to your GOLO Diet and exercise plan by acknowledging your efforts and accomplishments.

You'll develop a well-rounded strategy for attaining your weight reduction and fitness objectives by designing your workout program to work in conjunction with your GOLO Diet plan.

Finding joy in your physical activities will make the trip more pleasurable and sustainable.

Bear in mind that consistency and balance are vital.

You'll soon notice the benefits of mixing a nutritious diet with regular exercise for a healthier and more vibrant life if you are persistent and patient.

MAINTAINING YOUR PROGRESS AND EMBRACING A HEALTHIER LIFESTYLE

Building Lasting Habits for Continued Success

The secret to long-term success on the GOLO Diet is consistency.

You can lay a strong foundation for ongoing advancement and long-term wellbeing by adopting healthy practices into your daily routine.

Here are some techniques for creating enduring habits that will contribute to your ongoing success:

1. **Start little**: Start with little, doable adjustments. It might be daunting and unsustainable to try to completely change your way of life all at once.

Concentrate on one or two modest habits at a time, such as increasing your water intake or increasing the amount of veggies you eat at each meal.

2. **Set Achievable Goals**: Establish measurable objectives that can be achieved in a fair amount of time. Having specific goals can help you stay motivated and feel successful as you meet each milestone.

3. **Establish a Routine**: Set up a daily schedule that incorporates self-care activities, your GOLO Diet plan, and regular exercise.

Your ability to stay on track and regularly make better decisions is aided by having a scheduled schedule.

4. **Monitor Your Progress**: Log your food consumption, exercise routine, and other healthy behaviors in a journal or with an app. Maintaining accountability and spotting areas for development are both made possible by tracking your progress.

5. **Honor Your Successes**: Honor your accomplishments, no matter how minor. Reward and acknowledge yourself for adhering to your objectives and forming healthy habits.

Celebrating your accomplishments will encourage you to keep going and will reinforce the behavior.

6. **Embrace Mindfulness**: Throughout the day, be conscious of your decisions and actions. Pay attention to how your body is feeling and how certain foods and activities affect your overall health.

Making deliberate decisions that support your objectives can be facilitated by mindfulness.

7. **Surround Yourself with Support**: Discuss your objectives and advancement with encouraging friends, family members, or a partner in accountability.

Having a support network can offer inspiration, direction, and comprehension through trying times.

8. **Get Ready for Challenges**: Plan ahead for probable roadblocks and difficulties that may appear along the way.

Make a plan for how you will respond to these circumstances so that you are ready to continue on your path despite obstacles.

9. **Learn from Mistakes**: Making mistakes or experiencing setbacks is common. Consider them an opportunity to learn and grow rather than a reason to be disappointed.

Find out what caused the setback, then utilize it as a lesson to steer clear of it in the future.

10. **Exercise Patience and Perseverance**: Creating long-lasting habits requires time, and development may not always be linear. Be kind to yourself and persevere even when things seem to be moving slowly.

Keep in mind that even the smallest advancements will help you succeed in the long run.

It takes time to develop enduring habits, but with perseverance, consistency, and a positive outlook, you can design a lifestyle that supports your ongoing success with the GOLO Diet and beyond.

Celebrate your successes, embrace the journey, and keep in mind that the long-lasting adjustments you make now will pave the way for a healthier and happy tomorrow.

Overcoming Challenges and Staying Motivated on the GOLO Diet

Any diet plan you choose to follow will have its own set of problems.

This is also true of the GOLO Diet.

You can overcome these challenges and maintain your motivation on your path to greater health and well-being, though, if you have the correct attitude and tactics.

Here are some pointers to help you keep motivated and on track:

1. **Have Realistic Expectations**: Recognize that weight loss might not occur as rapidly as you'd want because progress takes time.

Instead of obsessing about the number on the scale, set reasonable expectations and concentrate on the wonderful improvements you are making.

2. **Adopt a growth mindset**: See obstacles as chances for development and education. If you run into obstacles or setbacks, view them as chances to get better and change your strategy rather than reasons to give up.

3. **Put Your Attention on Non-Scale Victories**: Celebrate non-scale successes like higher energy, a better mood, better sleep, or improved fitness. These beneficial modifications are equally significant signs of your GOLO Diet progress.

4. **Discover Your "Why"**: Recall the motivation behind your first decision to begin the GOLO Diet. Find your underlying reasons for wanting to get healthier and draw encouragement from them when things get tough.

5. **Establish a Support System**: Surround yourself with people who are understanding of and supportive of your aspirations. Inform those around you about your journey so they may offer support and hold you accountable.

6. **Prepare Ahead for Temptations**: Consider scenarios, such social gatherings or special occasions, where you might feel tempted to deviate from your GOLO Diet plan. Make better decisions in advance, or bring a dish that is GOLO-friendly to share.

7. **Practice Mindfulness**: Pay attention to your thoughts and feelings as you eat. Be conscious of emotional eating triggers and pay attention to your body's signals of hunger and fullness.

Making decisions that are in line with your objectives might be aided by mindfulness.

8. **Monitor Your Progress**: Log your meals, workouts, and other healthy routines in a journal or using an app. Monitoring your development helps keep you inspired and point out trends or potential improvement areas.

9. **Reward Yourself**: Honor your successes and advancements, no matter how minor. As a way to appreciate your effort and commitment, treat yourself to incentives that are not food-related.

10. **Be Kind to Yourself**: Keep in mind that everyone's journey to wellness includes highs and lows. If you have a setback, be kind to yourself and refrain from criticizing yourself. Make the most of setbacks to develop and learn.

11. **Change Up Your Routine**: Try out new dishes, experiment with various forms of exercise, or find fun methods to stay active to avoid being stuck in a rut.

Boredom can be avoided and engagement maintained via variety.

12. **Visualize Success**: Imagine attaining your goals and the wonderful effects it will have on your life. Visualization may boost your willpower and keep you focused on the right direction.

You can achieve long-term success and drastically improve your health and way of life by conquering obstacles and remaining motivated while following the GOLO Diet.

Never forget that development is made in even the smallest of steps.

Maintain your commitment, practice self-compassion, and have faith in your capacity to change for the better in order to achieve a healthier and happier future.

FREQUENTLY ASKED QUESTIONS ABOUT THE GOLO DIET

Addressing Common Concerns and Misconceptions

The GOLO Diet may cause confusion and inquiries, as with any diet or lifestyle change.

By addressing these worries, you can gain clarity and have the ability to decide on your health with knowledge.

Here, we address some common worries and misunderstandings about the GOLO Diet:

The GOLO Diet: Is it a Fad?

The GOLO Diet is not a trendy eating plan. It is a weight loss strategy based on research that emphasizes balanced diet, portion control, and keeping blood sugar levels consistent.

Instead of advocating short-term remedies, the program wants to encourage long-term, sustainable lifestyle improvements.

2. Does the GOLO diet necessitate calorie counting?

In contrast to other diets, the GOLO Diet places more emphasis on a special "Metabolic Fuel Matrix" than on calorie counting.

It promotes eating meals that are balanced in terms of protein, fat, and carbohydrates to maintain blood sugar levels and enhance metabolism.

3. Could Nutrient Deficiencies Occur Due to the GOLO Diet?

The GOLO Diet offers a balanced combination of nutrients from whole foods when it is properly followed.

To achieve your nutritional demands, you must, like with any diet, make sure you eat a variety of foods. A licensed dietician is a good resource for tailored advice.

4. Will the GOLO Diet Still Allow Me to Enjoy Carbohydrates?

Yes, carbohydrates in the form of entire, nutrient-dense foods like fruits, vegetables, whole grains, and legumes are permitted on the GOLO Diet.

The significance of selecting complex carbs versus refined and processed ones is emphasized.

5. Can Anyone Follow the GOLO Diet?

The GOLO Diet is typically regarded as secure and suitable for most people. Individual demands and health situations can, however, differ.

FREQUENTLY ASKED QUESTIONS ABOUT THE GOLO DIET

Before beginning any new diet or fitness regimen, it is imperative to seek medical advice, especially if you have any particular health issues or diseases.

6. Will the GOLO Diet Cause Me to Lose Weight Quickly?

Results for weight loss might vary depending on a number of variables, including starting weight, metabolism, and program adherence.

While some people may lose weight quickly, others might do so more gradually.

The GOLO Diet encourages long-term success above short-term outcomes by emphasizing sustained weight loss.

7. Can I Follow the GOLO Diet Without Any Restrictions?

The GOLO Diet encourages portion control and mindful eating even though it offers a flexible approach to eating.

Even when eating healthier foods, overeating might thwart weight loss goals. Balance and moderation are crucial elements of the program.

8. Do Expensive Supplements Need to Be Taken with the GOLO Diet?

The GOLO Diet includes supplemental products that are optional but may improve metabolic health; they are not necessary for program success.

Instead of supplements, the emphasis is primarily on complete, healthy foods.

Keep in mind that every person will have a different experience with a diet, so it's important to pay attention to your body's needs.

You can make knowledgeable choices regarding the GOLO Diet and modify the method to suit your unique needs by addressing your worries and misconceptions.

Consider speaking with a licensed dietitian or healthcare expert who can help you on your path to wellness for individualized counsel.

EXPERT INSIGHTS AND TIPS FOR OPTIMIZING YOUR GOLO EXPERIENCE

We've gathered expert thoughts and advice to help you get the most of your GOLO Diet experience in order to ensure your success and happiness:

1. **Seek Professional Advice:** Consulting with a Registered Dietitian or Healthcare Professional can provide individualized guidance and ensure that the GOLO Diet corresponds with your unique health needs and goals.

2. **Adopt a real-foods diet**: Put an emphasis on including entire, nutrient-dense foods in your diet.

To provide your body the nutrition it needs, choose lean meats, fruits, vegetables, whole grains, and healthy fats.

3. **Maintain Proper Hydration**: Good hydration is crucial for general health and wellbeing. To boost weight loss attempts, energy levels, and digestion, consume lots of water throughout the day.

4. **Make sleep a priority**. Aim for seven to nine hours of good sleep each night. Regulating hormones, metabolism, and supporting your entire GOLO Diet experience all depend on getting enough sleep.

5. **Engage in Mindful Eating**: Pay attention and be present when you eat. You may notice hunger and fullness cues, stop overeating, and improve your appreciation of food by practicing mindful eating.

6. **Be Patient and Consistent**: Long-term weight loss requires patience. Maintain your patience and perseverance, and try not to let brief setbacks demotivate you. Think about the advancements you're making.

7. **Pay attention to how various foods and activities make you feel by listening to your body**. Your body offers insightful input to direct your decisions and enhance your GOLO experience.

8. **Exercise Regularly**: Include regular exercise in your routine to promote weight loss, increase fitness, and improve general wellbeing.

9. **Manage Stress**: Look for healthy methods of stress management, such as yoga, meditation, or time spent in nature. Chronic stress can have an influence on health in general and weight loss.

10. **Establish Achievable and reasonable Goals**: Prioritize reasonable goals for your GOLO Diet journey. Celebrate each accomplishment and keep in mind that progress is a gradual process.

11. **Don't Make Comparisons**: Concentrate on your own development rather than making comparisons to others. Everybody's journey is different, and your accomplishments are worthwhile.

12. **Maintain a Positive Attitude**: Develop a positive view and confidence in your capacity for success. You can maintain motivation and conquer obstacles by adopting a positive mindset.

13. **Recognize and Celebrate Non-Scale Victories**: Highlight non-scale triumphs like more vigor, a happier mood, or better sleep. These are significant

markers of your development.

14. **Continue Your Education**: Keep up with the latest information on diet, exercise, and health. Knowing more enables you to make wise selections and change your strategy as necessary.

15. **Enjoy the Process**: Take pleasure in your path toward better health. Keep in mind that the GOLO Diet promotes complete well-being in addition to weight loss.

You may create a good and rewarding journey toward greater health and long-lasting lifestyle improvements by incorporating these professional insights and advice into your experience with the GOLO Diet.

Maintain your dedication, enthusiasm, and faith in your capacity to reach your health objectives.

Keep in mind that over time, even the smallest advancements add up to big gains.

CONCLUSION: EMBRACE THE GOLO DIET FOR SUSTAINABLE WEIGHT LOSS

Recap of Key Takeaways

Let's review some key insights from our investigation into the GOLO Diet and celebrate the success stories of those who have adopted this method of promoting health and wellbeing.

Key Learnings:

1. **Nutritionally Balanced Meals**: The GOLO Diet places a strong emphasis on meals that combine protein, lipids, and carbohydrates.

Putting an emphasis on complete, nutrient-rich foods helps to maintain stable blood sugar levels and advances general health.

2. **Metabolic Fuel Matrix**: The "Metabolic Fuel Matrix," which promotes portion control and attentive consumption of particular food types to improve metabolism, is the focus of the GOLO Diet rather than monitoring calories.

3. **Exercise and Activity**: Regular exercise is crucial for fitness, weight loss, and general wellbeing. The route to health is improved by including an active lifestyle into the GOLO Diet.

4. **Mindful Eating**: Mindful eating encourages a deeper connection with food and aids in limiting excess. Eating mindfully encourages healthier decisions and supports a pleasant connection with food.

5. **Individualized Approach**: The GOLO Diet can be modified to fit a person's preferences and needs. The plan will be in line with specific health objectives if qualified dietitians or other medical specialists are consulted.

SUCCESS STORIES

1. **Sarah**: Sarah found the GOLO Diet after battling with yo-yo dieting and became disillusioned with unsustainable weight loss strategies.

She lost weight steadily and increased her overall energy by following the program's balanced strategy and including frequent exercise.

Sarah was proud of her mental and emotional improvements in addition to her physical changes.

2. **Mike and Lisa**: Mike and Lisa made the decision to start their health journey together as a pair.

They discovered that because of the GOLO Diet's focus on real, whole foods, planning and preparing meals was fun.

By encouraging one another and sticking to their healthy routines, Mike and Lisa were able to celebrate significant weight loss and felt closer as a couple.

3. **James**: James was looking for a holistic approach to better his health because he struggled with emotional eating and a sedentary lifestyle.

He was able to address his emotional triggers and establish a healthier connection with food because to the GOLO Diet's emphasis on mindfulness.

James lost a significant amount of weight and developed a deeper sense of self through consistent exercise and the encouragement of his GOLO group.

These success stories demonstrate how the GOLO Diet can enable people to accomplish their weight loss and health objectives.

People can experience both physical improvements and positive changes in their overall well-being by adopting balanced diet, mindful eating, and an active lifestyle.

The GOLO Diet is a potential option for people looking to improve their health and happiness over the long run since it provides a sustainable and individualized approach to wellness.

Keep in mind that every person's road to wellness is different, making it crucial to choose a strategy that speaks to you personally.

Put your health first, enjoy the trip, and recognize your accomplishments as you go—whether you choose the GOLO Diet or another way of living.

I wish you health and happiness!

YOUR PATH TO A HEALTHIER AND HAPPIER YOU!

Congratulations for starting the path to a healthier and happier version of yourself! Remember that this is a revolutionary process that goes beyond simply reducing weight as you adopt the GOLO Diet's principals and move toward healthy lifestyle adjustments.

To achieve holistic wellbeing, you must nurture your body, mind, and spirit. Here are some motivating words to help you along the way:

1. **Celebrate Every Step Forward, No Matter How Small**: Be fair to yourself and embrace progress rather than perfection. Recognize that change takes time and that each healthy decision you make improves your wellbeing as a whole.

2. **Experience the Joy of Movement**: Being active need not be a chore. Find things to do that make you happy and feel alive. Moving your body should be enjoyable, whether you're dancing, hiking, or attempting a new sport.

3. **Nourish Your Body**: Pay attention to giving your body the nutrition it needs to be healthy and to give you energy. Enjoy the flavors of whole, natural foods and be grateful for the health benefits they provide for your body.

4. **Develop Mindfulness**: A wonderful tool for aware life is mindfulness. Being

in the moment helps you understand your body's demands, choose meals carefully, and manage stress.

5. **Look for Community and Support**: You don't have to do this journey alone yourself. Be in a supportive environment, whether it be friends, family, or others that share your viewpoints and are traveling a similar journey. You may support and inspire one another by working together.

6. **Remain Committed to Your Goals**: It's common to run into obstacles and failures, but don't allow that stop you from pursuing your objectives. Keep working toward your objectives and never forget that every day presents an opportunity to make wise decisions.

7. **Find equilibrium**: Make an effort to maintain equilibrium in every area of your life. Maintain a healthy balance among your everyday activities, exercise, and meals. Create a sense of balance in your life that fosters wellbeing in all areas.

8. **Honor Non-Scale Wins**: Keep in mind that success is measured by more than just weight. As you move along your path, enjoy the enhancements in your energy, mood, and general health.

9. **Love Yourself**: Practice self-acceptance and love for yourself. Your value is not determined by how you look or by a scale number. As you proceed on your journey to a better you, be kind and loving to yourself.

10. **Make It a Lifelong Journey**: Happiness and health are constant goals. Recognize that this is a lifelong journey as you make progress. Accept the growth process, and keep changing, adapting, and learning.

Your journey to a healthier, happier version of yourself is individual and full of opportunities for personal development.

Remember to treasure each step of your life-changing adventure as you adhere to the GOLO Diet's tenets and adopt healthy routines.

Recognize that you have the power to improve yourself and have faith in your capacity to bring about positive change.

Accept this route with an open mind and a firm dedication to your wellbeing.

Here's wishing you a bright, healthy, and happy future!